The impact

Soua Goumou

The impact of the Ebola epidemic on HIV PMTCT

Prevention of mother-to-child transmission of HIV from 2013-2016 in the N'zérékoré region, Republic of Guinea

ScienciaScripts

Imprint

Any brand names and product names mentioned in this book are subject to trademark, brand or patent protection and are trademarks or registered trademarks of their respective holders. The use of brand names, product names, common names, trade names, product descriptions etc. even without a particular marking in this work is in no way to be construed to mean that such names may be regarded as unrestricted in respect of trademark and brand protection legislation and could thus be used by anyone.

Cover image: www.ingimage.com

This book is a translation from the original published under ISBN 978-3-639-52537-3.

Publisher:
Sciencia Scripts
is a trademark of
Dodo Books Indian Ocean Ltd. and OmniScriptum S.R.L publishing group

120 High Road, East Finchley, London, N2 9ED, United Kingdom
Str. Armeneasca 28/1, office 1, Chisinau MD-2012, Republic of Moldova, Europe

ISBN: 978-620-6-08134-0

Table of contents :

SUMMARY

The N'Zérékoré region has 6 health districts with a total population of 1,696,807 in 2015 [1]. HIV prevalence is 1.6% in Guinea, with 120,000 people including 65,000 women [2]. During the Ebola epidemic in Guinea, the N'Zérékoré region was the most affected, resulting in dysfunctional health services. The aim of this study was to assess the impact of the Ebola epidemic on HIV PMTCT. It covered a 4-year period and focused on HIV-positive pregnant women and their children in 19 health centers. We found a prevalence rate of 0.88% and an acceptance rate of 44.03%. Housewives accounted for 64%. The ARV treatment completion rate fell from 54.95% to 23.23%. The number of people lost to follow-up increased during the Ebola epidemic. On the other hand, the rate of assisted deliveries fell from 94.87% to 69.17% p = 8.126e-06. Similarly, the number of children protected decreased from 50.55% to 16.67%. HIV PMTCT has been negatively impacted, as evidenced by the drop in the number of assisted deliveries, the increase in the number of lost to follow-up, break-

ups, etc...

I. INTRODUCTION

The N'Zérékoré region is one of eight administrative regions of the Republic of Guinea, bordered to the south by Liberia and Sierra Leone, to the east by the Ivory Coast, to the north by the Kankan region and to the west by the Faranah region. The total population is estimated at 1,696,807 hbt in 2015 [1]. The region is culturally and ethnically diverse. Between 1990 and 2003, the region experienced very significant migratory movements. The climate in the N'Zérékoré region is hot and humid, alternating between an eight-month rainy season and a dry season that lasts only four months, which is favorable to tropical diseases.

According to UNiCEF, in 2014 national HIV prevalence was 1.6% among adults, an estimated 120,000 people living with HIV, including 65,000 women [2]. The N'Zérékoré region borders one of the countries with high prevalences in the West African sub-region (Ivory Coast 3.5% with 250,000 women). For several years now, a number of health structures/services have included PMTCT activities in their minimum package of activities (PMA).

From December 2013 to March 2016, West Africa experienced the largest and longest-running Ebola epidemic in human history, with over 28,000 cases and more than 11,000 deaths (situation as of September 2015). In addition to the three hardest-hit countries of Liberia, Guinea and Sierra Leone, cases have been reported in Nigeria (20 cases / 8 deaths), Mali (8 cases / 6 deaths), Senegal (1 case / 0 deaths) and the USA (4 cases / 1 death). Spain, Italy and Great Britain each reported one case of the disease [.3] In Guinea, it was the health districts of the N'Zérékoré region that paid the heaviest price during the Ebola epidemic. There were 742 cases in Macenta, with a case-fatality rate of 66%, 381 cases in Gueckédou, with a case-fatality rate of 75%, and 254 cases in N'Zérékoré, with 65% deaths [4].

The Ebola virus disease was little known to health workers and communities alike. The similarity of certain signs of Ebola virus disease to those of malaria (fever, headache, vomiting, etc.) made people afraid to use health services for fear of being mistaken for Ebola patients. This situation of psychosis has considerably reduced the number of people using the services of the various programs.

Since the end of the Ebola epidemic, very few studies have been carried out to assess the impact of the epidemic on the evolution of various health programs. And no studies have been carried out on HIV, particularly on the prevention of mother-to-child transmission of HIV in the N'Zérékoré region, the area hardest hit by the epidemic. This lack of information on PMTCT of HIV motivated us to choose "The impact of the Ebola epidemic on PMTCT of HIV in the N'Zérékoré region of Guinea" as our Master's thesis, in order to understand what had happened and contribute to improving PMTCT of HIV.

1.1. Research question

What impact has the MVE epidemic had on the Prevention of Mother-to-Child Transmission of HIV?

1.2. Objectives

1.2.1 . General objective :

Assess the impact of the Ebola epidemic on the Prevention of Mother-to-Child Transmission of HIV.

1.2.2 Specific objectives:

❖ Determine the proportion of pregnant women tested for HIV before, during and after the Ebola epidemic.

❖ Estimating HIV prevalence among pregnant women before, during and after the Ebola epidemic

❖ Determine PMTCT drop-out rates before, during and after the Ebola epidemic.

❖ Determine the proportion of unassisted deliveries of children of HIV-positive mothers before, during and after the Ebola virus disease epidemic.

❖ Compare indicators (HIV test acceptance rate, treatment adherence rate, PMTCT dropout rate, number of days out of medication, number of assisted deliveries, number of children correctly monitored) from the periods before, during and after the Ebola virus disease epidemic.

1.3. Research hypotheses

Was there a decrease in the use of PMTCT services during the epidemic?

Was there an increase in the number of people losing their sight during the epidemic?

Was there an increase in the risk of mother-to-child transmission during the epidemic period?

II. METHODOLOGY

2.1. Study framework

Our study took place in the N'Zérékoré region, which has 6 health districts (N'Zérékoré, Lola, Macenta, Gueckedou, Yomou and Beyle); 6 hospitals, including 01 regional; 77 integrated health centers; 201 integrated health posts and 60 non-integrated health posts, 03 communal medical centers or integrated improved health centers for public facilities. The situation for private facilities is as follows: 20 private pharmacies, 8 faith-based facilities, 5 dispensaries. Of these, 41 offer PMTCT activities, 19 of which were visited during the course of the study. (See attached list).

2.2. Type and duration of study

This is a historical cohort, covering the period from January 01, 2013 to December 31, 2016 taking into account the presence of the Ebola virus disease epidemic. (Before, during and after)

- Previously: January to December 2013

- During: January 2014 to December 2015

- After : January to December 2016

2.3. Target population

Our study targeted HIV-positive women in the N'Zérékoré region. We were interested in pregnant women who consulted and/or were registered in the 19 structures offering HIV PMTCT activities.

2.4. Study population

The study involved women whose files were available and correctly completed at the time of our visit.

2.5. Sampling

We carried out purposive sampling oriented towards facilities that had started HIV PMTCT in 2013.

2.6. Data collection and analysis

2.6.1. Individual data collection form: a survey form was drawn up containing all the study variables (explanatory variable, variables to be explained).

2.6.2. Data collection: three health workers were trained in data collection and took part in the process.

ANC consultation registers, ANC sheets, mother and child follow-up sheets, PMTCT monthly reports, input stock sheets, etc. ...

1.3.1 Data analysis: data were entered into Excel 2013 and EPIDATA, then exported to R statistical software for analysis,

2.7. Variables definition

2.7.1 Taking ARVs

Complete ARV treatment: treatment started in 14ème S with compliance during pregnancy and at birth.

Incomplete intake: started treatment on time but did not finish, or lost sight of, or started after 28ème S.

No intake: who did not receive ARVs during pregnancy.

2.7.2 Start of treatment

Early onset: started at 14ème weeks or before 28ème

Late intake: from week 28 ^{ème}

2.7.3 Number of visits

Number of scheduled medical visits: number of visits required during a pregnancy in an HIV field.

Number of medical visits respected: number of visits carried out

2.7.4 Children's serological status

HIV-negative: negative HIV test

Seropositive: positive HIV test

2.7.5 Birth

Delivery mode: vaginal delivery, Caesarean section

Place of delivery

-structure: follow-up health structure

-At home: outside care structures and without assistance.

other structure: health structure different from that of follow-up

2.7.6 HIV-positive woman: woman with a positive HIV strip test,

*2.7.7. Test positive***:** test with a dash in the patient field and a dash in the control field.

Child status : Alive, deceased; transferred; lost to sight.

*Protected child***:** child whose mother started treatment at 14ème weeks, who has respected all follow-up appointments, who has taken ARVs in full and correctly, who has given birth in a qualified facility, received prophylaxis at birth and whose baby has benefited from ARV prophylaxis.

2.8 Ethics: we requested authorization from the regional health directorate to collect and use data from the region's PMTCT. The survey forms are anonymous, and once the collected data have been entered, they are archived in a locked, secure cabinet.

III. RESULTS

1.1 Socio-professional characteristics of HIV-positive pregnant women in the Nzérékoré region from 2013 to 2016.

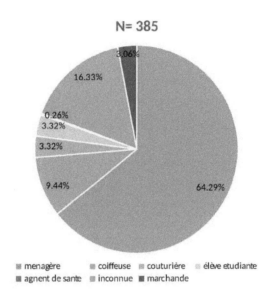

Figure 1: Socio-professional characteristics of HIV-positive pregnant women in the Nzérékoré region from 2013 to 2016.

In the population of HIV-positive pregnant women who consulted in the Nzérékoré region between 2013 and 2016, 64% [95% CI 59.22-68.80] were housewives, 17% [95% CI 13.25-20.75] women of unknown profession, 10% [95% CI 7-13] hairdressers and 3% [95% CI 1.29-4.71] for each of the following three professions: hairdresser, student or pupil and merchant. (See Fig. 1). The distribution of HIV-positive pregnant women according to occupation is identical for both rural and urban areas in the Nzérékoré region of Guinea. $X^2 = 9.78$, ddl = 6, p-value = 0.1344. We found that 78% [95% CI 73.83-82.17] of women lived in urban areas versus 22% in rural areas. As for their ages, the average was 26 years [95% CI 25.43-26.57], with extremes ranging from 15 to 49 years. The mean age distribution of pregnant women was identical in all three study periods. (Kruskal-Wallis = 1.0357, ddl = 2,p = 0.5958).

1.2 Monitoring women in the presence of the Ebola virus epidemic

Table 1: Distribution of HIV-positive women from 2013 to 2016 according to

Nzérékoré region and presence of the Ebola Virus Disease

epidemic

Districts	Before (2013)	For (2014-2015)	After (2016)	Total
Beyla	4	0	3	7
Gueckedou	22	21	51	94
Lola	0	6	1	7
Macenta	15	18	27	60
N'zerekore	43	45	81	169
Yomou	7	4	36	47
	91(23.70%)	94 (24.48%)	199 (51.82%)	384(100)
Total	[73.83-82.17]	[20.16-28.79]	[46.84-56.80]	

Between 2013 and 2016, 119,897 pregnant women consulted for CPN1 in 19 structures in the region and 52786 agreed to be tested, an overall acceptance rate of 44.03%.

Of the pregnant women tested, 464 were diagnosed HIV-positive, with a prevalence of 0.88% IC95% [0.79-0.96%]. Of the 464 HIV-positive pregnant women, 384 had documented follow-up, giving an effective follow-up rate of almost 83% IC95% [79.36-86.22%].

Among them, 91 pregnant women, or 23.70% of women, were monitored in2013 before the outbreak of the epidemic.

From 2014 to 2015, i.e. during the two-year Ebola epidemic, the number dropped to 94 pregnant women, or 24.48%. And during the first post-Ebola year, 199 women tested positive and were followed up in the 19 Centers visited during our study in the Nzérékoré region, representing nearly 52% of the total number of HIV+ women followed up. (See table 1). The proportions of HIV-positive pregnant women followed up in the 19 centers visited in the region differ according to the presence of the epidemic $X^2 = 34.06$, $ddl = 10, p = 18.0710^{15}$.

1.3 . Taking ARVs by HIV-positive women during PMTCT

Table 2: *distribution of ARV intake by pregnant women during PMTCT in the N'Zérékoré region between 2013-2016.*

Taking ARVs		FrequenciesProportions
Complete	12131	.67%IC$_{95\%}$ [27.00-36.33]
Incomplete plug	23361%	[56.12-65.88]
Catch in progress		225.76% [3.43-8.09]
Without socket		61.57% [0.32-2.82]
Total	382100%	

Table 3: *Distribution of complete ARV intake by women pregnant during PMTCT in the N'Zérékoré region between 2013- 2016.*

Full course of ARVs

Periods	No	Yes	Total
Before	41	50 (54.95%)	91
For	68	25 (26.88%)	93
After	152	46 (23.23%)	198
Total	261	121(31.67%)	382

$X^2 = 30.277$, ddl= 2, p= 2.663e-07

In the 19 HIV PMTCT structures we visited, 121 women took their ARV treatment correctly and completely (see table 2). Before the start of the Ebola epidemic, 50 (54.95%) of the 91 women we monitored were able to take their treatment correctly and completely. During the two (2) years of the MVE epidemic, out of 94 HIV-positive pregnant women monitored, only 25 (26.88%) took their ARVs correctly. And in the "post-Ebola" period, 23.23% took their ARVs in full in the first year. The differences in the proportions taking ARVs in full observed between the periods (Before, during and After) are statistically significant. $X^2 = 30.277$, ddl = 2, p= 2.663e-07. The age distribution according to ARV intake shows that the mean age is identical in the intake groups. (Kruskal-Wallis chi-squared = 2.2739, ddl = 5,p = 0.8101)

3.4 Situation of those lost to follow-up during HIV PMTCT

Table 4: *Distribution of follow-up status of pregnant women* *during PMTCT in the N'Zérékoré region between 2013-2016.*

Follow-up status	Frequencies	Proportion (%)
Complete	230	60.21
Lost from sight	88	23.04
Refusal	3	0.78
Follow-up in progress	22	5.76
No follow-up	39	10.21
Total	382	100

Table 5: *Breakdown of women lost to PMTCT by period (before, during and after)*

Periods	Lost from sight		Total
	No	Yes	
Before	81	10(11%)	91
For	72	22(23.40%)	94
After	141	56(28.43%)	197

| Total | 294 | 88 (23.04%) | 382 |

$X^2 = 10.685$, df $= 2$, p $= 4,8$ W^3

During the 4 years covered by our study, 60.21% of HIV-positive women followed up in the 19 health centers reached the end of their follow-up, compared with 23.04% who were lost to follow-up and 10.21% not followed up (see table 4).

The proportion of HIV-positive pregnant women lost to follow-up differs according to the period (before, during and after).

$X^2 = 10,685$, ddl $= 2$, p $= 4.8$ W^3 . (See Table 5).

3.5 Assisted childbirth for children of HIV-positive mothers on ARVs.

Table 6: *Distribution of deliveries of children by women on ARVs in the N'Zérékoré region between 2013-2016.*

Assisted childbirth

Periods	No	Yes	Total
Avant(2013)	4	74 (94.87%)	78
During (2014-	9	65 (87.84%)	74
2015)			
After (2016)	37	83 (69.17%)	120
Total	50	222 (81.61%)	272

$X^2 = 23.441$, ddl= 2, p-value = 8.126e-06

The proportion of assisted deliveries fell from 94.87% before the Ebola EVD epidemic to 69.17% in the post-Ebola period. During the two years of the Ebola EVD epidemic 65 deliveries were assisted, i.e. a rate of 87.84% for 2014 and 2O15.The difference in proportion observed is not due to chance, it is statistically significant with $X^2 = 23.441$, df = 2, p-value = 8.126e-06. (Table 6).

3.6 Children protected by HIV PMTCT activities

Table 7: *Distribution of children born to HIV-positive mothers according to PMTCT HIV protection in the N'Zérékoré region between 2013- 2016.*

Protected children

Periods	Yes	No	Total
Before	46 (50.55%)	45	91
For	17 (18.28%)	75	93
After	33 (16.67%)	164	198
Total	96 (25.26%)	284	380

$X^2 = 40.62$, ddl = 2,p = 1.512e-09

To better understand the impact of the Ebola epidemic on the outcome of PMTCT in children, given that the tests at 6eme weeks and 18eme months are not practically done. We created a "protected child" variable: a child whose mother started treatment at 14eme weeks, who respected all follow-up appointments, who took ARVs in full and correctly, who gave birth in a qualified facility, received prophylaxis at birth and whose baby benefited from ARV prophylaxis. This analysis shows that the proportion of protected children fell from 50.55% before the MVE epidemic to 16.67% in the post-Ebola period. During the two years of the epidemic, only 17 children, or 18%, were protected (see table 7). This difference in the proportion of children protected is highly significant with $X^2 = 40.62$, ddl= 2,p = 1.512e-09

3.7 Place of delivery for children of HIV-positive mothers

Table 8: *Distribution of HIV-positive women by place of delivery in the Nzérékoré region from 2013 to 2016.*

	Frequency	Percentage
Delivery sites		
Follow-up structure	169	62.13

Home	49	18.01
Hospital	49	18.01
Private clinic	4	1.47
Health center	1	0.37
Total	272	100

62.13% of women followed up to delivery gave birth in their follow-up facility, 18% in hospital and at home, and 1.47% in private facilities. (Table 8). When these proportions are spread over the study period, we see that there is a statistically significant difference in proportion with $X^2 = 57.247$, ddl= 8,p= 1.612e-09

3.8 Trends in HIV PMTCT indicators in the Nzérékoré region between 2013 and 2016.

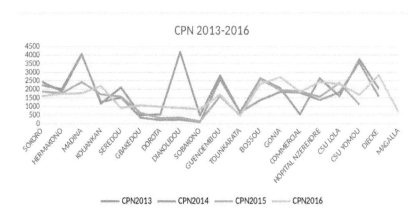

Figure 2: Trends in ANC between 2013-2016 in structures visited

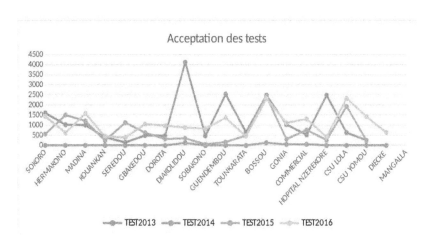

Figure 3: Trend in acceptance of HIV tests between 2013-2016 in

structures visited

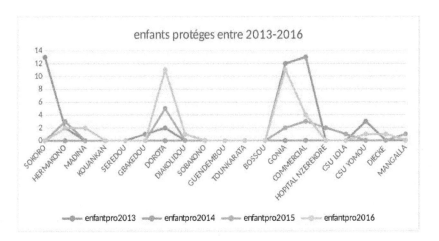

Figure 4: *Trends in ANC between 2013-2016 in structures visited*

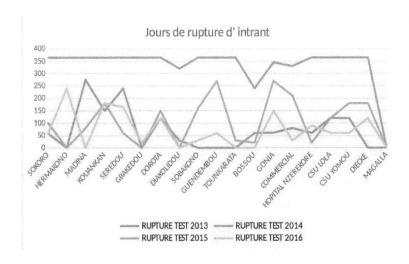

Figure 5: *Trend in days of input(test) shortages between*

20132016 in structures visited

Table 9: *Trends in PMTCT indicators in the Nzérékoré region*

from 2013 to 2016.

Indicators	Before (2013)	During (2014-2015)	After (2016)
Number of CPN	36024	52937	30936
Test acceptance rate	56.40%	23.73%	63.17%
Incidence	5.36 ‰	8.67 ‰	13‰
Children monitored	75/109	63/109	78/246
	(68.81 %)	(58.80%)	(31.71%)
Children tested 6ème S	0	0	0
Children tested at 18ème M	0	0	3
proportion		17/92(18%)	
of protected children	46/91		33/197
	(50.55 %)		(16.67%)
Number of days of break	1376	8379	1380

HIV prevalence in FE	0.88%

The acceptance rate for the screening test fell from 56.40% in the pre-Ebola period to 23.73% during the epidemic, then rose to 63.17% in the first year after Ebola. (See fig.3). HIV diagnosed in pregnant women rose from 5.36‰ to 13‰ between 2013 and 2016. Testing of children at 6eme weeks and 18eme months remains unperformed in the Nzérékoré region.

The proportion of children protected has fallen considerably from 50.55% in 2013 (Before the epidemic), to 18% for both 2014 and 2015 and 16.67% in 2016. (Table 8 and 9).

ARV coverage among pregnant women in the N'Zérékoré region between 2013-2017 was 98.43% and 95.75% among children of HIV-positive mothers.

In the 19 structures of the 6 Health Districts of the N'Zérékoré region, there is at least one health worker trained in HIV PMTCT who worked during the period covered by our study.

IV. DISCUSSION

We have an HIV prevalence of 0.88% in the population of pregnant women in the N'Zérékoré region between 2013 and 2017. This prevalence is lower than the national prevalence of 2.5% found by ENSS in 2008 [8]. It is also lower than the 3.66% prevalence found by DAINGUY ME et Coll. in 2014 at BONOUA Hospital in Côte d'Ivoire[7] . We found that housewives are the most affected with 64% [95% CI 59.22-68.80], this trend could be explained by the low level of education of most of them. They are followed by hairdressers with a proportion of 10%. These results are contrary to those of Serge C et al. in Cameroon, who had 15.5% hairdressers, followed by secretaries (14.8%) [5] . The rate of acceptance of the test by pregnant women fell considerably from 56.40% in the pre-Ebola period to 23.73% during the epidemic, then rose to 63.17% in the first year after Ebola.

As for the follow-up rate of women, it increased considerably during the study period from 23.70% to 52%. This increase is statistically significant $p = 18.07\ 10^5$ and is due to the improved availability of tests and inputs from 2015 onwards. The completion of ARV treatment by pregnant women was negatively influenced by the presence of the MVE epidemic (p= 2.663e-07). Indeed, we found a significant increase in the proportion of women lost to follow-up during the epidemic ($p = 4.8\ 10^{-3)}$). Similarly, the proportion of assisted deliveries fell from 94.87% to 94.87%.

before the MVE epidemic to 69.17% in the post-Ebola period (p = 8.126e-06). We also found that the proportion of protected children decreased from 50.55% before the MVE epidemic to 16.67% in the post-Ebola period (p = 1.512e-09). A Delamou et Coll study on the effects of the MVE epidemic on maternal and child health found a decrease in the number of prenatal consultations, vaccination coverage and the number of assisted deliveries.

The decline in the various indicators is thought to be due to rumours linked to the Ebola Virus Disease, which led to a lack of confidence and fear of being considered as an MVE suspect. The number of deaths in the communities, and even of health workers and the approaches used during interventions, have provoked strong reluctance on the part of the population.

Overall ARV coverage among pregnant women in the N'Zérékoré region between 2013-2017 was 98.43% and 95.75% among children of HIV-positive mothers. These rates are 17% and 15% respectively at national level [8]. The number of days of disruption increased during the crisis, particularly in 2014, when HIV PMTCT activities were not carried out due to the total disruption of inputs. This break was due to the fact that all actors had directed their support towards the Ebola response.

Testing of children born to HIV-positive mothers at $6^{\text{ème}}$ weeks and $18^{\text{ème}}$ months was not carried out in the Nzérékoré region during the period under review.

On the other hand, in the 19 facilities in the 6 health districts of the N'Zérékoré region, there was at least one health worker trained in HIV PMTCT who worked during the period covered by our study.

CONCLUSION

Our objective was to assess the impact of the MVE epidemic on the prevention of mother-to-child transmission (PMTCT) of HIV in the N'Zérékoré region. The results of the analysis and field observations show that PMTCT of HIV was negatively impacted by the MVE health crisis, as evidenced by a drop in the number of children protected, an increase in the number of days when PMTCT inputs were unavailable, a drop in the rate of acceptance of screening tests by pregnant women, an increase in the number of women lost to follow-up, a drop in the number of women attending ANC and a drop in the number of assisted deliveries.

ACKNOWLEDGEMENTS

I give glory to God for giving me the health and ability to follow and complete this SPSD Master's degree.

I would like to thank the teaching staff at the University of Aix-Marseille for the quality of the courses given, the experiences shared and their availability over the years.

I would also like to thank my local referees Dr KISI MUNDIETE Adrien and Dr CAMARA Alioune as well as my mentor Dr SOULA Georges for their support during the preparation of the dissertation.

I can't finish without thanking the Francophonie, the University of Aix-Marseille and the Conseil Santé for their technical, financial and material support during the training and work placement.

REFERENCES

[1] *RapportEDS-MICS 2012*, ICF International and Institut National de la Statistique (INS), BP 221, Conakry, Guinea. Available at www.stat- guinée.org

[2] **Unicef: State of The World's Children 2016 Country Statistical Information** Accessible at: *www.unicef.org/french/infobycountry/guinea_statistics.html* page consulted on 09 /12/ 2016.

[3] **Lars H, Hannover L MG, Hannover D. Don't be too quick to claim victory.** *Swiss Medical Forum* 2015 ;15(47) : 1094-1096

[4] **Fond Mondial. Poverty Reduction Strategy Paper (PRSPIII 2013-2015), Guinea July 2013 Accessible at** *https://www.imf.org/external/french/pubs/ft/scr/2013/crl3191f.pd f* 12/25/2016

[5] Serge C , Billong RF, Samuel MS, Mosoko JJ, Gabriel LE, Bissek ACZ, Bosco N E. Epidemiological distribution of HIV infection among pregnant women in the ten regions of Cameroon

and strategic implications for prevention programs, *PafMed J.* 2015; 20:79 doi:10.11604/pamj.2015.20.79.42

[6] World AIDS Day 2011 Report. Geneva, UNAIDS, 2011 available *at* http://poledoc.bibli.fr/opac/doc num.php?explnum id=348 25/12/2016

[7] DAINGUY ME, KOUAKOU C, KOUADIO E, TRABI G, GRO BI A, DJIVOHESSOUN A, DJOMAN I FOLQUET AM; prevention of mother-to-child transmission (ptme) in a semi-rural Ivorian setting: experience of bonoua general hospital Rev int sc méd 2014;16,3:181-186.

[8] PROGRAMME NATIONAL DE PRISE EN CHARGE SANITAIRE ET DE PREVENTION DES STI/VIH/SIDA ; Normes et Procédures en Prévention de la Transmission Mère Enfant du VIH - PTME GUINEE, AOUT *2013. PP 6*

[9] A Delamou MD, S Sidibe MD, S D Sandouno MD); A Delamou, S Sidibe, B S Camara MD, A H Beavogui, A MEl Ayadi ScD, T Delvaux PhD, Prof V De Brouwere PhD; J

Okumura PhD, W H Zhang PhD; Effect of Ebola virus disease on maternal and child health services in Guinea: a retrospective observational cohort studywww.thelancet.com/lancetgh Published online **February 22, 2017** *http://dx,doi.org/10.1016/S2214-109X(17)30078-5*

15/03/2017

Mailing address

DrGOUMOUSoua, Physician

Yattaya/ C Ratoma/ Conakry

Tel:+224 622 476 692

Email : souagoumou@gmail.com

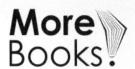
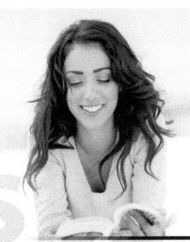

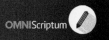